Constipation

How To Treat Constipation
How To Prevent Constipation
Along With Nutrition, Diet, And Exercise For Constipation

By Ace McCloud
Copyright © 2013

Disclaimer

The information provided in this book is designed to provide helpful information on the subjects discussed. This book is not meant to be used, nor should it be used, to diagnose or treat any medical condition. For diagnosis or treatment of any medical problem, consult your own physician. The publisher and author are not responsible for any specific health or allergy needs that may require medical supervision and are not liable for any damages or negative consequences from any treatment, action, application or preparation, to any person reading or following the information in this book. Any references included are provided for informational purposes only. Readers should be aware that any websites or links listed in this book may change.

Table of Contents

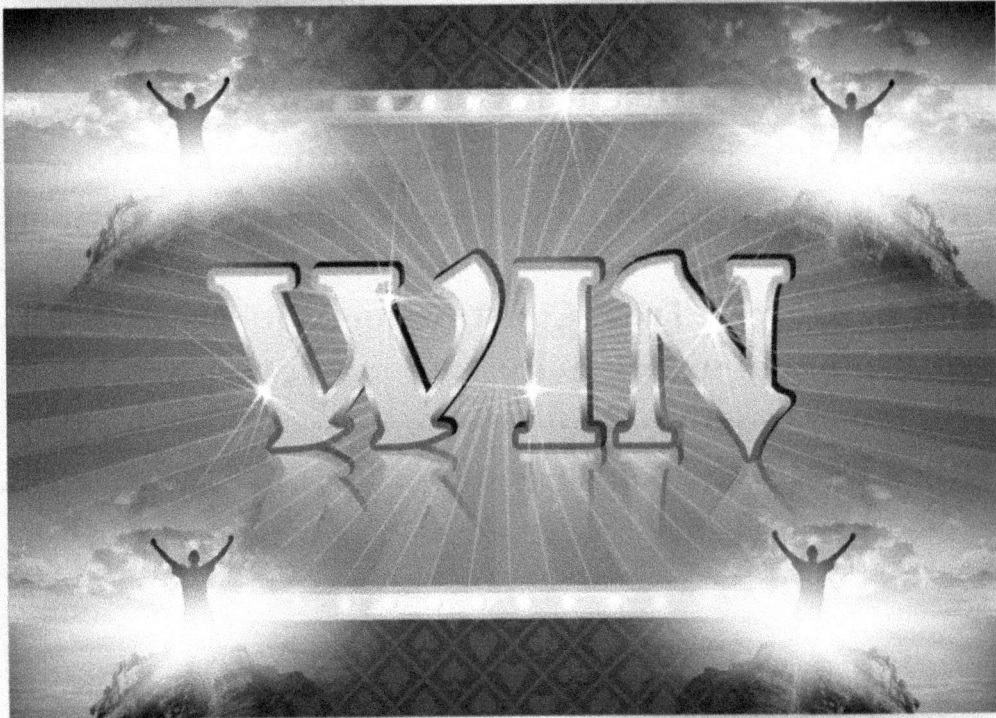

Be sure to check out my website for all my Books and Audio books.

www.AcesEbooks.com

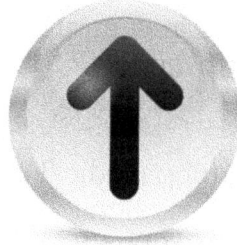

Introduction

I want to thank you and congratulate you for buying the book, "Constipation: How To Treat Constipation- How To Prevent Constipation- Along With Nutrition Diet And Exercise For Constipation."

This book contains proven steps and strategies on how to deal with being constipated, as well as a general overview of the condition and how to prevent constipation from occurring in the first place.

While generally not a life-threatening medical condition, constipation can cause large amounts of physical discomfort, along with feelings of embarrassment and uneasiness. Just know that if you suffer from constipation, you are not alone, and that this book can serve as your all-inclusive reference on how to prevent and treat constipation through diet, lifestyle choices, natural remedies, and modern medicine.

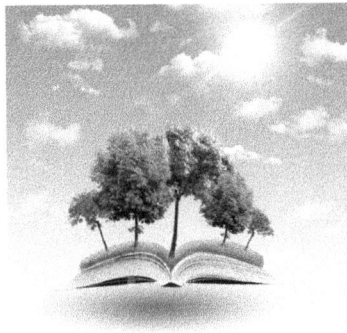

Chapter 1: Overview of Constipation

The term "constipation" is used to refer to the digestive condition of individuals who are experiencing a significant decrease in defecation frequency, incomplete bowel evacuation during bowel movements, and/or difficulty or intense straining during bowel movements. It is diagnosed in those who have bowel movements fewer than 3 times per week, and can be associated with extreme pain during defecation, as well as extremely hard stool.

Constipation is a fairly common issue for millions, and generally does not turn into a serious medical disorder. However, in certain cases, it can lead to other hazardous complications, such as hemorrhoids.

Chronic constipation can lead to obstipation, which results in the complete failure to pass any stool or gas. Also a potential health risk, fecal impaction can lead to complete bowel obstructions for long periods of time, which can become a life-threatening condition if left untreated.

While both men and women suffer from the condition, women seem to be slightly more at risk, especially due to hormonal changes during pregnancy. Also, older adults experience constipation more than middle-aged individuals.

Chapter 2: Causes of Constipation

Given that constipation is a symptom, and not a medical disease or disorder itself, the underlying cause of the constipation must be dealt with in order to alleviate the symptoms.

Causes of constipation fall into two general categories: obstructed defecation and colonic slow transit constipation (also referred to as hypomobility). While mechanical and functional problems are at the root of obstructed defecation, colonic slow transit constipation is caused by more external factors.

Foods

While an overall lack of fiber and extreme dehydration are usually the main dietary culprits of constipation, there are certain foods that are known to complicate bowel movements in certain individuals. Red meats like pork and beef, though extremely tasty, are difficult for the body to digest, and can cause constipation. Sugary products like cakes, pastries, pies, and cookies are also extremely delicious. However, these items tend to be low in fiber, and over-consuming them can lead to constipation. Dairy products also tend to be low in fiber and high in saturated fats, and can not only put you at risk of constipation, but of heart diseases as well. Processed food items such as pizza, pasta, frozen dinners, and instant mashed potatoes tend to make constipation worse, as they are extremely low in fiber. Finally, caffeine's dehydrating quality can greatly increase your risk for constipation. Consumers of excessive amounts of coffee, chocolate, and tea should be wary of developing constipation.

Medications

Among the medications known to bring about constipation are pain medications such as Tylenol and Percocet, antidepressants such as Elavil and Tofranil, anticonvulsants such as Dilantin and Tegretol, and aluminum-containing antacids such as Amphojel and Basaljel. Iron supplements are also believed to cause the side effect of constipation.

Medical Conditions

Certain medical conditions can also cause constipation. Parkinson's disease, depression, diabetes, thyroid disease, and stroke, to name a few, are all believed to cause constipation. In addition, hormonal disturbances, such as an underactive thyroid gland, can lead to constipation.

Heavy Metals

It's also a good idea to monitor your body's levels of heavy metals, such as mercury and lead. These types of metals have also been linked to constipation.

Voluntary Constipation

For some individuals, the cause of their constipation is purely psychological. They may be germaphobes and have a fear of using public restrooms, have a fear of the pain they have been experiencing recently during defecation, or just decide to hold it in for one reason or another.

Chapter 3: How To Diagnose Constipation

The diagnosis of constipation is generally made from a patient's description of their bowel movements. The revealing characteristics are frequency of bowel movements, difficulty and pain in passing stool, consistency of stool, bloating, headaches, feeling of fatigue, and incomplete bowel movements.

Dietary Habits And Medical Condition

Speaking to a patient about their dietary habits and medical situation will also offer some clues as to whether conditions for constipation are present. Any indication of low fiber intake, low amounts of hydrating fluids, or consumption of medications associated with constipation are clear signs that that the person is at a high risk of being constipated.

Rectal Exam

For a more certain diagnosis, a qualified medical professional may need to inspect a patient's rectal area, focusing on whether the lower rectum has traces of feces or not. Inspecting stool can give a better idea of stool consistency, the presence of hemorrhoids and/or blood, and whether the patient has any abnormalities in that area. A physician may perform the examination by hand, or may make use of a colonoscope.

X-Rays

Taking x-rays of the abdominal area can give medical staff a clear picture of the intestinal tract, but are generally only taken if bowel obstruction is suspected. However, x-rays are extremely useful, as they may reveal large amounts of fecal matter in the colon.

Irritable Bowel Syndrome (IBS)

For patients experiencing chronic constipation symptoms for at least 3 days each month for more than 3 consecutive months with no obvious cause, a diagnosis of irritable bowel syndrome (IBS) may be given.

Severe Defecatory Dysfunction (SDD)

In very rare cases, an individual may be experiencing constipation due to abnormal wave sequences in the colon. These cases are referred to as severe defecatory dysfunction (SDD), and have been recently treated successfully using nerve stimulation.

Chapter 4: How To Prevent Constipation

Preventing constipation is much easier (and far less uncomfortable) than treating it. Additionally, preventing constipation through proper diet, adequate exercise habits, and sufficient fluid intake, among other things, can save individuals the trouble of having to take medications or undergo procedures farther down the road.

Diet High In Fiber

The proper diet to prevent constipation should be very high in fiber. Fiber-rich foods are extremely helpful in preventing constipation because they act as natural laxatives, helping the colon cleanse itself of fecal matter. Doctors and nutritionists recommend at least 25 to 50 grams of fiber each day in order to ensure healthy bowel movements.

Foods High In Fiber

Foods that are high in fiber include apples, bananas, chickpeas, lentils, beans, raspberries, blueberries, cabbage, carrots, whole grain bread, oats, whole wheat and rye flours, wheat germ, wheat bran, and figs.

Perhaps the most effective food of all to relieve constipation is prunes. Prunes contain very high amounts of dietary fiber, and are such an effective laxative that doctors usually recommend drinking prune juice to treat constipation naturally.

Be cautious, though, not to increase your fiber intake too quickly, as it may cause bad gas or diarrhea.

Metamucil

Metamucil is a fiber supplement (also known as a bulk laxative) that can help promote healthier bowel movements. Just be sure to take it with plenty of water. Also, taking too much of supplements like this over long periods of time can actually cause constipation, so don't overdo it.

Herbal Laxatives

Along with preventing constipation, many herbs can act as appetite stimulants, can strengthen the stomach, and can promote healthy digestion. Among the herbs you might want to try are Ginger, Buckthorn, Senna, Rhubarb, Cascara Sagrada, and Aloe Vera. Senna works particularly well in tea form and is extremely powerful! A nice glass of Senna Tea along with a large glass of water afterwards can help alleviate even the most stubborn of constipations. A great Senna Tea Product is: Smooth Move Senna Tea. It is best only to take these herbs when needed, as over time the body can become reliant on these herbs for constipation relief if they are over used.

Probiotics

Probiotics are live microscopic organisms that are naturally present in the digestive tract and aid with digestion. Probiotics help in preventing constipation by limiting the growth of harmful bacteria, improving immune function, enhancing the digestive tract's protective barrier, and promoting the production of vitamin K. A great Probiotic that I personally use every day is: PB 8 Probiotic.

Folic Acid

Aside from the foods mentioned previously, you may want to consider taking folic acid, which is known to help prevent constipation. Folic acid is contained within most multivitamins, or can be taken on its own. A great Folic Acid supplement is: Now Foods Folic Acid.

Apple Pectin

Along with eating apples, individuals looking to ward off constipation may want to consider adding apple pectin to their diet. Apple pectin is a compound found in many apples, along with other fruits, such as apricots, cherries, and citrus peels. Not only can it be used to help move things along in the digestive tract, but it can also be ingested to help harden stool for people with diarrhea. The substance is available at health food stores, or carried in the vitamin aisle at major grocery chains. A great ApplePrectin Supplement is: Now Foods Apple Pectin.

Lots Of Water

To keep your intestines well lubricated, doctors recommend drinking at least 8 cups of water every day. Along with its lubricating qualities, water keeps the food in your digestive tract moist, allowing it to be passed during bowel movements more easily. My favorite way to get pure clean water at a good price is with: ZeroWater and ZeroWater Replacement Filters.

Exercise

Exercising regularly is another great and easy way to prevent constipation. Being physically active stimulates the intestinal muscles, enabling them to work more efficiently and effectively. Plus, frequent exercise lowers the time required for food to pass through your intestinal tract. As a result, stool retains more moisture and remains softer, making bowel movements less difficult.

Any type of aerobic exercise (such as running, jogging, or swimming) can help keep the digestive tract working properly. But even walking for 10 to 15 minutes several times per day will aid the digestive system.

Yoga

The soothing and relaxing qualities of yoga make it a very effective method for preventing constipation, as yoga lowers blood pressure and relieves stress. There are specific poses, however, which lend themselves to preventing constipation.

The first pose is called baddha konasana. While sitting on the ground, bring the soles of your feet together, and let your knees drop as far towards the ground as you can. Pull your heels in as close to your groin area as possible. Then, wrap your hands around your feet, sit up nice and tall so that your spine is straight, and relax your shoulders. Flutter your knees up and down to loosen your lower area. If you are limber enough, lower your face down to the ground, keeping your hands on your feet and your back straight. Hold the position for 5 to 10 breaths, and then roll yourself back to the upright position, repeating as needed.

The second yoga pose you can try is called ardha matsyendrasana. Sitting on the ground, cross your right foot to the outside of your left thigh. If you don't feel limber enough, place the right foot on the inside of the left thigh. Once you are comfortable, arch your left toes back towards you, so you feel a pull in your left calf area. Then, hook your right arm in front of your right knee, and turn to look back over your left shoulder. Remember to inhale and exhale deeply, and keep your spine straight. Hold for 5 to 10 breaths, and then repeat on the other side.

The third yoga position is referred to as pavanamuktasana, and is also known as the 'wind relieving pose.' Lying on your back, bring your right knee up towards your chest, keeping your left leg pressed down on the ground. Flex your toes back towards you, keeping your calf area tight. Continue bringing your right knee up higher, relaxing the right hip area as you do so. Hold for 5 to 10 breaths, and then repeat on the other side.

A fourth yoga position you can try is called halasana. Laying on your back, bring both legs up over your head and place them behind you, with only your feet touching the ground. Your entire lower and middle back should be up off the ground, and you should be supporting yourself with your hands resting on your lower back, and your upper arm laying flat on the ground. Hold for 5 to 10 breaths, and then, still keeping your spine straight, bring your legs back out in front of you.

The final yoga pose you can try to help prevent constipation is called savasana. Lay on the ground in a very relaxed position, with your legs spread shoulder width apart, and your arms away from your body. Your fingers and toes should be completely limp, and your palms facing upward. Close your eyes, and concentrate on relaxing all parts of your body, especially the abdominal area. Hold for 5 to 10 breaths.

Low Stress Levels

Reducing stress levels is also a very effective way to prevent constipation, as mental stress has a huge effect on how well your bowel functions. Given that bowel movements depend on complex signal mechanisms sent from your brain, it makes sense that when your brain is under duress; your bowel is as well. Also, when people are more stressed, they are less likely to exercise, and more likely to binge on unhealthy foods, further increasing their risk of constipation.

Don't Ignore Bowel Movement Urges

To keep your bowels functioning properly, it's important to pay attention to your body's internal clock. Don't ignore the urges from your body telling you that it's time to defecate. The longer you wait to go, the more water is extracted from your stool, which will make the stool harder to pass. While you don't have to commit to having a bowel movement at the exact same time every day, give yourself enough time during your morning, afternoon, or evening routine so that you don't feel like you have to hold it until you have more free time to go.

Give Children Frequent Bathroom Breaks

For children especially, be sure to give them scheduled toilet breaks throughout the day. At the very least, they should be brought to the bathroom in the early morning, 30 minutes after every meal, and before bed. Often times, children will say that they do not need to go, simply out of embarrassment or a desire to not want to stop the fun activity they may be participating in. But requiring them to physically go to the bathroom periodically will encourage them to use the toilet, and not voluntarily hold in their bowel movements.

Prepare For Travel

Finally, be especially mindful of developing constipation when you are on the go. Traveling makes people even more pressed for time, as they need to rush to catch trains, planes, buses, and taxis to make it to business meetings, conferences, and events. Make sure you remember to hydrate frequently while waiting for connecting transportation, and to pack fresh fruits, dried figs and prunes, granola bars, and trail mix when you know you will be out all day. And don't forget to throw some workout gear into your suitcase, so that you can maintain your healthy lifestyle, even on the road.

Chapter 5: All Natural Remedies For Treating Constipation

If you are wary of taking medications, there are plenty of all natural remedies you can try to help relieve your constipation. For pregnant women especially, a natural remedy offers the benefits of treating the condition without the potential side effects associated with many medications.

While some ingredients may not be conveniently available at your local supermarket, there are plenty of health food stores and health-related websites out there for you to purchase hard-to-find items.

Triphala Powder

Triphala powder is a mix of three medicinal plants: amla, myrobalan, and belleric myrobalan. It is a very popular laxative in the Indian culture, and helps with regulating digestion and bowel movements. To prepare, either add one teaspoon to warm water or mix with honey and eat. Consuming triphala powder once per day on an empty stomach (either first thing in the morning or before bed) can help relieve constipation very quickly. A great product is: Organic India Triphala Powder.

Raisins

Raisins are packed with tons of fiber, and act as a fantastic natural laxative. To soften them up a bit, you can soak a handful overnight in water, and eat them first thing in the morning while your stomach is still empty.

Guavas

The guava fruit has lots of fiber in the pulp and seeds. Also, guava contributes to mucus production in the anus, and aids in peristalsis, the contractions along the intestinal tract that help push ingested food out of the body.

Lemon Juice

To deal with constipation, drink a warm glass of water mixed with one teaspoon of lemon juice and a pinch of salt first thing in the morning. It not only will help cleanse your intestines, but will assist with the easy passage of stool.

Figs, Dates and Prunes

Dried or fresh figs are a great source of fiber, and can work wonders in relieving constipation. Before bed, boil a couple of figs in some milk, and drink the mixture while it is still warm. Dates and prunes also work great, and can be prepared in the same manner.

Flax Seeds

Flax seeds also contain a great deal of fiber. Since they taste a bit bland, try adding them to your morning cereal, or eat a handful with warm water at breakfast. A great brand of Flaxseed is: Bob's Organic Whole Flaxseed.

Castor Oil

A timeless natural remedy, castor oil is great for treating constipation, and can also kill intestinal worms. If the taste bothers you, add a tablespoon to a warm glass of milk, and drink it before bed. A great Castor Oil is: Now Foods Castor Oil.

Spinach

Spinach is a nutrient-packing veggie that can cleanse and rebuild the intestinal tract. Cooking spinach is extremely easy, and simply requires steaming it for a couple of minutes. However, when trying to treat constipation, taking spinach on its own is the most effective way. Twice a day, mix 100 mL of spinach juice with 100 mL of water and drink.

Oranges

While most people think of Vitamin C when they think of oranges, the juicy citrus fruit also contain large amounts of fiber. Try eating two oranges each day (once in the morning and once in the evening) to provide relief for your constipation.

Seed Mixtures

Along with flax seed, there are other seeds that can be used to treat constipation. Mix some sunflower seeds, flax seeds, sesame seeds, and almonds together, grinding them to a fine powder. Eat one tablespoon of this mixture everyday for a week to help eliminate your constipation. You can eat it by itself, or mix it in with salads or cereals. Not only will it deal with your constipation, but the mixture will help rejuvenate your intestinal walls.

Grapes

Grapes are a great natural laxative, as they contain large amounts of cellulose, natural sugars, and other organic material that can help with constipation. Try eating at least 350 grams of grapes each day while you are constipated to relieve symptoms.

Bael Fruit

The bael fruit is considered the best of all natural laxatives, and is also an effective way to tone up a person's intestines. In addition, eating it regularly for 2 to 3 months will help clean out old and accumulated fecal matter.

Licorice

Chewing a couple of licorice sticks every day can be very helpful in treating constipation, as licorice is a wonderful natural laxative.

Psyllium Husk

Each night before going to bed, add 3 teaspoons of psyllium husk to a cup of warm milk or water, and drink. A great brand of Psyllium Husk is: Now Foods Psyllium Husk.

Beans

Some great beans to add to your diet include kidney beans, soy beans, navy beans, chick peas, and lentils.

Brown Rice

Lastly, try switching brown rice for white rice during your lunch and dinner meals. Brown rice contains more fiber, and is therefore more effective in treating constipation.

Juicing and blending

Juicing and blending are also excellent and highly recommended ways to relieve constipation. Just juice or blend your favorite fruits and vegetables along with some of the ingredients mentioned above. Some other good fruits that are good for constipation and that can be juiced or blended are berries, peaches, apricots and plums. If your constipation isn't too serious, you will be regular before you know it. An incredible juicer is the: Breville Juice Fountain and a great Smoothie Blender is the: NutriBullet Blender. A smoothie of fruits and vegetables in the morning along with a large glass of water, followed by a long walk is a great recipe to get some fairly quick relief!

Prune Juice

One of the best ways to relieve constipation naturally or prevent it from occurring is simply with a glass of prune juice followed by a large glass of water.

Acupuncture

Aside from consuming all natural dietary items, you may want to consider acupuncture. Acupuncture is a traditional healing process that involves applying pressure with your fingers to specific pressure points on the body. Large

Intestine 4 is a pressure point that many acupuncturists believe to be associated with constipation, as well as other internal organs. It is located at the highest point of the muscle that connects the thumb to the forefinger.

While acupuncture is much safer than other modern medical procedures, there are certain side effects that you may experience. Fatigue, soreness, bruising, muscle twitching, and lightheadedness are all possible side effects of acupuncture.

Hypnosis

Finally, if you suffer from constipation, you might want to try hypnosis. All parts of the body, including the bowel area, are controlled by signals sent from the mind. Hypnosis can communicate with your unconscious mind and get it to properly control the digestive and excretion processes, thereby alleviating you of your constipation. My favorite place to get Hypnosis is at: Hypnosis Downloads.

Chapter 6: How To Treat Constipation With Modern Medicine

If you wish to take medication to relieve your constipation, there are plenty of FDA-approved drugs (and even some procedures) that have proven themselves to be very effective. Keep in mind, however, that all drugs, prescription or otherwise, may cause harmful side effects, and be sure to be on the lookout for active ingredients you may be allergic to. Be sure to consult with a physician before starting on any medication, and have them monitor your status regularly so that other harmful conditions do not develop.

Furthermore, medication laxatives should not be used as a long-term strategy to deal with constipation. You don't want your body to get into the habit of depending on these substances to complete the excretion process, further weakening your already malfunctioning digestive system. Use them as a last resort, as it is generally best to deal with your constipation issues through diet and lifestyle changes.

In extreme cases, your doctor may suggest performing a procedure to help with your constipation. But again, every effort should be made to treat your constipation through diet and lifestyle changes.

Correctol

Correctol is a stimulant that causes rhythmic contractions in the intestinal tract. These contractions aid the stool in passing through the body more smoothly. Side effects may include abdominal discomfort, nausea, and cramps.

Colace

Colace falls under the category of 'stool softeners.' Stool softeners moisten the stool, and also help to prevent dehydration. Possible side effects include bloating, diarrhea, throat irritation, and nausea.

Milk of Magnesia

Milk of magnesia is a mix of magnesium hydroxide and water, and gets its name from its milk-like appearance (thought it is also available in tablet form). To relieve constipation, milk of magnesia acts like a sponge and draws water into the colon to help stool pass more easily. Along with constipation, it can be used to alleviate indigestion and heartburn. Side effects include diarrhea, loss of too much water, and body mineral imbalances.

Amitiza

Amitiza is approved by the FDA for treating chronic constipation from an unknown cause, as opposed to constipation due to another medical condition or medication. It softens the stool by increasing its water content, allowing the stool to pass more easily. Amitiza should be taken twice per day, with food. The side effects of this drug include headaches, nausea, diarrhea, abdominal pain, and vomiting.

Linzess

Linzess comes in capsule form, and should be taken once per day on an empty stomach. Be sure to take it at least 30 minutes prior to the first meal of the day. This drug helps ease constipation by aiding bowel movements in occurring more frequently.

While Linzess does not have a reputation for causing terrible side effects, it has been associated with diarrhea. Also, keep in mind that Linzess is not approved for patients under the age of 18.

Cephula

Cephula is a prescription laxative that operates by drawing water into the bowel to soften and loosen stool. Its common side effects include gas, diarrhea, upset stomach, and abdominal cramps.

Miralax

Miralax is highly recommended for patients who cannot tolerate dietary fiber supplements. It assists in producing softer stool by causing water to remain in the stool. Miralax Laxative Powder.

Disimpaction and Enema

If laxatives are not effective in breaking up your stool, a physician may perform a procedure called disimpaction. The physician will gently insert a gloved finger into your rectum to manually break up the stool. Then, a laxative enema will be administered (liquid squeezed into colon to bring about a bowel movement).

Surgery

Only in extreme cases will surgery be used to clear up constipation. During the surgery, medical professionals will remove part of your colon area, focusing on the problematic section of your anal sphincter or rectum. But again, surgery should be used only as a very last resort.

Conclusion

I hope this book was able to help you better understand the causes of constipation, and how to deal with constipation through diet, lifestyle choices, natural remedies, and medications.

The next step is to decide which form(s) of prevention or treatment is right for you. Remember that preventing constipation from occurring is much easier and less painful than dealing with the condition. Keep in mind that constipation is a very common issue for millions of people, so don't be afraid to talk to those around you and to seek out advice from those who have dealt with constipation before.

Finally, if you discovered at least one thing that has helped you or that you think would be beneficial to someone else, be sure to take a few seconds to easily post a quick positive review. As an author, your positive feedback is desperately needed. Your highly valuable five star reviews are like a river of golden joy flowing through a sunny forest of mighty trees and beautiful flowers! *To do your good deed in making the world a better place by helping others with your valuable insight, just leave a nice review.*

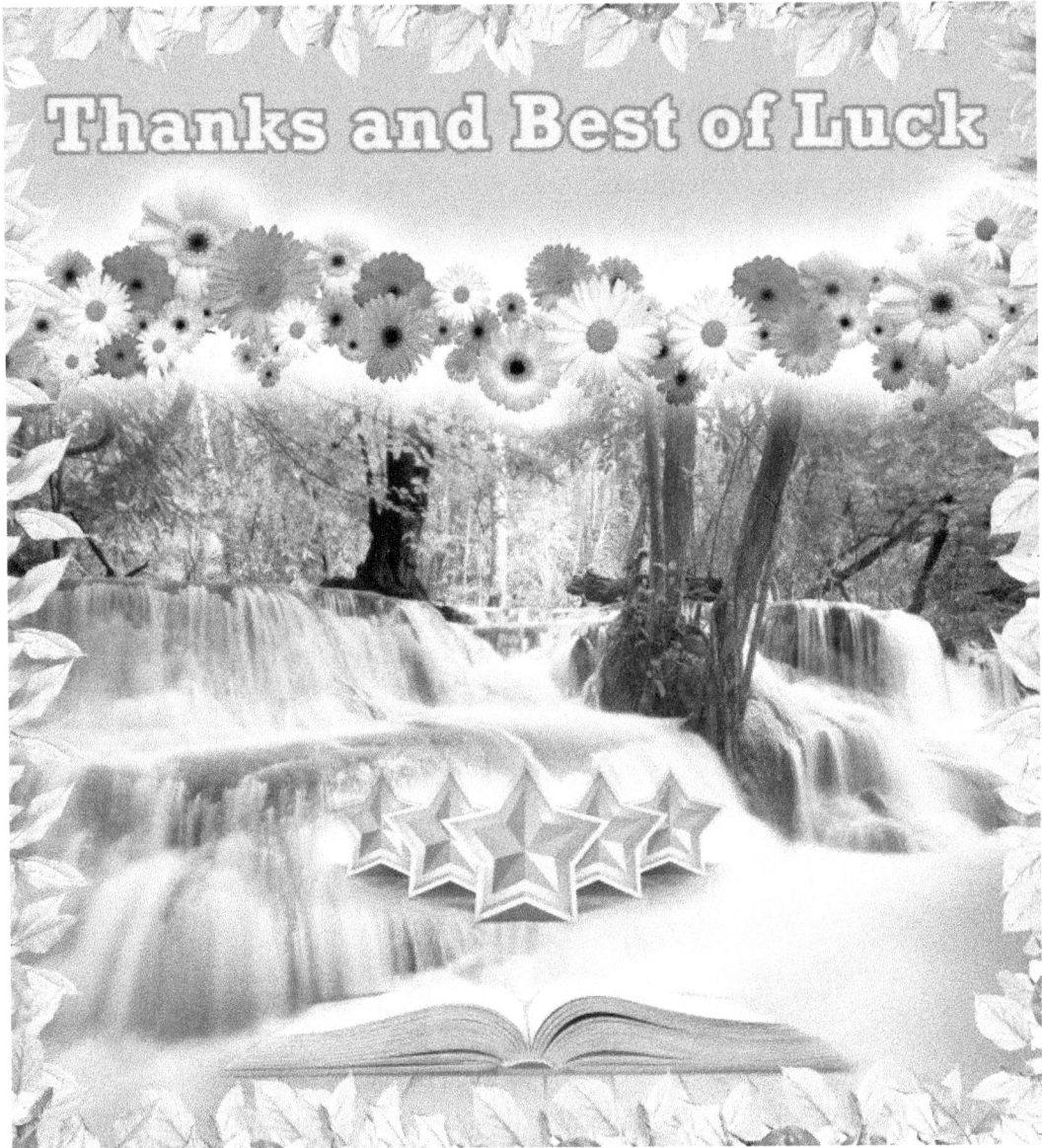

Thanks and Best of Luck

My Other Books and Audio Books

Health Books

ULTIMATE HEALTH SECRETS

HEALTH

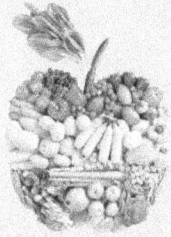

Strategies For Dieting, Eating Healthy, Exercising, Losing Weight, The Mediterranean Diet, Strength Training, And All About Vitamins, Minerals, And Supplements

Ace McCloud

ENERGY
ULTIMATE ENERGY

Discover How To Increase Your Energy Levels Using The Best All Natural Foods, Supplements And Strategies For A Life Full Of Abundant Energy

Ace McCloud

RECIPE BOOK

The Best Food Recipes That Are Delicious, Healthy, Great For Energy And Easy To Make

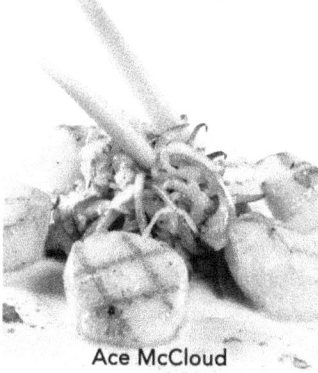

Ace McCloud

MASSAGE THERAPY

TRIGGER POINT THERAPY
ACUPRESSURE THERAPY
Learn The Best Techniques For Optimum Pain Relief And Relaxation

Ace McCloud

LOSE WEIGHT

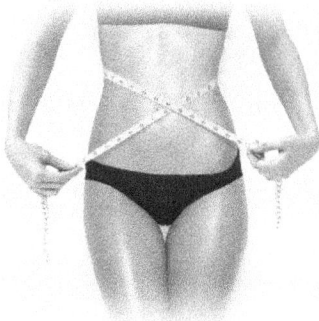

THE TOP 100 BEST WAYS TO LOSE WEIGHT QUICKLY AND HEALTHILY

Ace McCloud

FATIGUE
OVERCOME CHRONIC FATIGUE

Discover How To Energize Your Body & Mind So That You Can Bring The Energy & Passion Back Into Your Life

Ace McCloud

Peak Performance Books

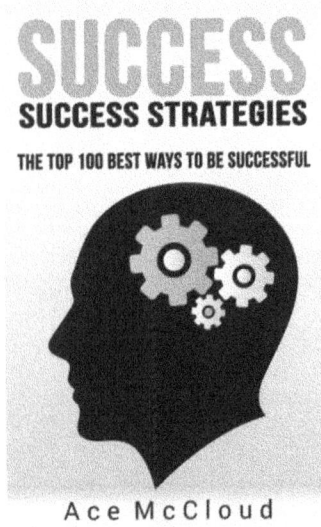

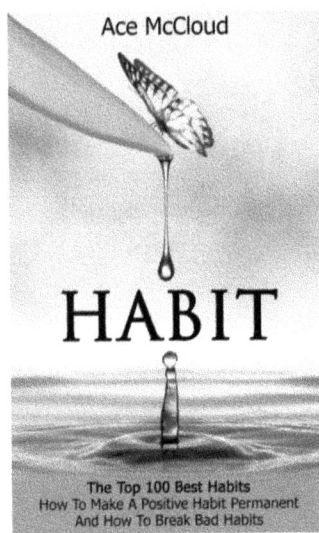

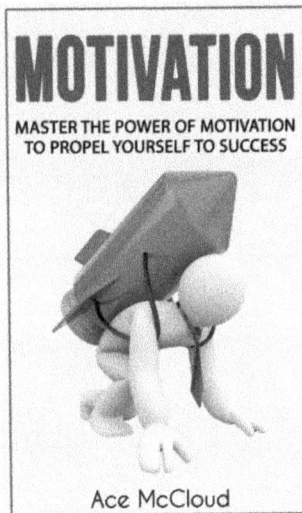

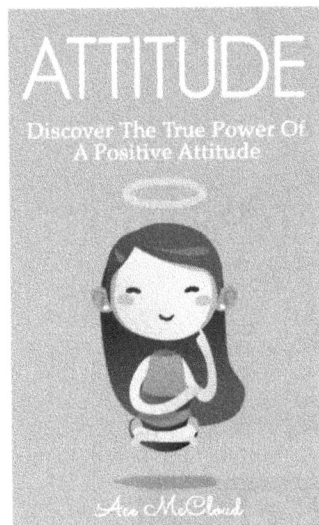

SUCCESS
SUCCESS STRATEGIES
THE TOP 100 BEST WAYS TO BE SUCCESSFUL

Ace McCloud

Ace McCloud

HABIT

The Top 100 Best Habits
How To Make A Positive Habit Permanent
And How To Break Bad Habits

MOTIVATION

MASTER THE POWER OF MOTIVATION
TO PROPEL YOURSELF TO SUCCESS

Ace McCloud

ATTITUDE

Discover The True Power Of
A Positive Attitude

Ace McCloud

SELF DISCIPLINE

Unleash The Power Of Self Discipline, Influence And Willpower In Your Life To Achieve Anything

Ace McCloud

Competitive Strategies

WINNING STRATEGIES

The Top 100 Best Strategies For Peak Performance During Competitions

Ace McCloud

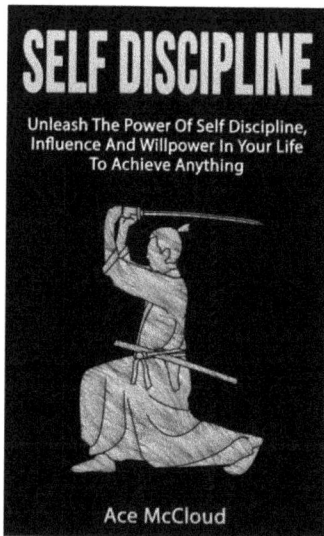

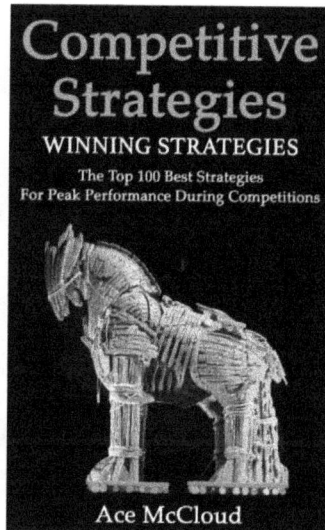

Be sure to check out my audio books as well!

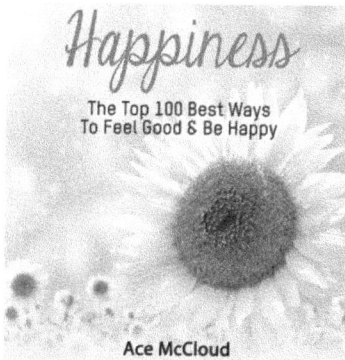

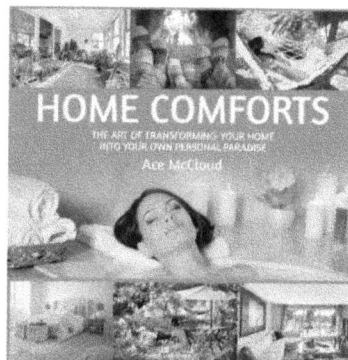

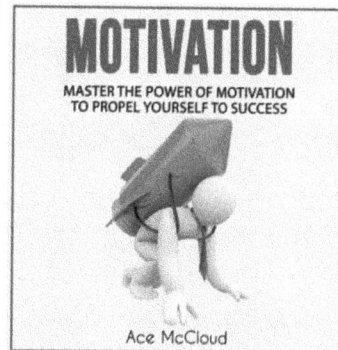

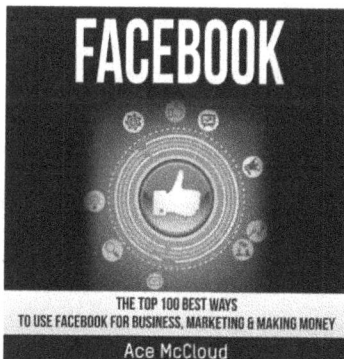

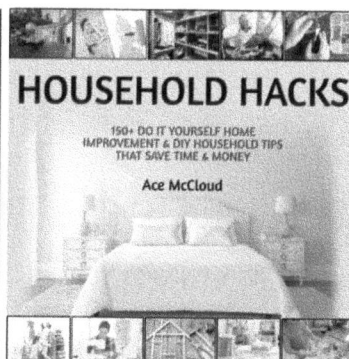

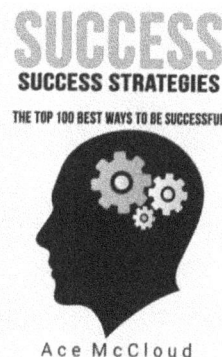

Happiness

The Top 100 Best Ways To Feel Good & Be Happy

Ace McCloud

HOME COMFORTS

THE ART OF TRANSFORMING YOUR HOME INTO YOUR OWN PERSONAL PARADISE

Ace McCloud

MOTIVATION

MASTER THE POWER OF MOTIVATION TO PROPEL YOURSELF TO SUCCESS

Ace McCloud

FACEBOOK

THE TOP 100 BEST WAYS TO USE FACEBOOK FOR BUSINESS, MARKETING & MAKING MONEY

Ace McCloud

HOUSEHOLD HACKS

150+ DO IT YOURSELF HOME IMPROVEMENT & DIY HOUSEHOLD TIPS THAT SAVE TIME & MONEY

Ace McCloud

SUCCESS

SUCCESS STRATEGIES

THE TOP 100 BEST WAYS TO BE SUCCESSFUL

Ace McCloud

Check out my website at: www.AcesEbooks.com for a complete list of all of my books and high quality audio books. I enjoy bringing you the best knowledge in the world and wish you the best in using this information to make your journey through life better and more enjoyable! **Best of luck to you!**